Home Doctor:

Heal Yourself Using Only Natural Herbs and

Oils. 70+ Recipes To Stay Healthy

Table of Contents

Introduction

Home remedies prove helpful to deal with lots of common and complex ailment. Luckily, there are numerous herbs that can be used to treat a number of ailments. Hiccups may be the most annoying and the funniest ailments.

Although these hiccups are not life threatening, they can still be annoying and cause discomfort. Hiccups usually result from many involuntary contractions of your diaphragm, which are the muscle between your abdomen and chest. Hiccups may be caused by misfired message from your brain that may get stuck in a continuously occurring loop.

The cure for hiccups is to swallow a teaspoon full of sugar, or you can even gargle with ice water for around 30 seconds. Hagen, a famous physician, says that both the tricks probably do send up a signal to your brain that may disrupt the message loop, which would allow your diaphragm to relax.

However, if your hiccups last for more than 48 hours or become severe that it is hard to eat or breathe, then you should contact a doctor. In rare cases, hiccups can be a symptom of brain injury, a stroke or even multiple sclerosis.

The cure for minor injuries is to place the small-burned area under running cold water for several minutes until all the pain has subsidies. This would also help to reduce the swelling. Then you should apply a thin layer of lotion that contains Aloe Vera a particular segment of an aloe leaf that is into cut lengthwise, which should be directly on the burn.

However, use takes caution when applying lotion to the potentially infected as it can seal in the infection and prevent proper healing. Hence, great care should be taken when healing with burns.

Congestion in chest and sneezing could result from a cold caused by some viral infection that may appear in your upper respiratory tract. The cure for cold and flu is simple that can be easily followed at home. A bowl of chicken soup is the best remedy to fight cold and flu.

Even onion and garlic stock in the broth have anti-inflammatory, and the steam of these herbs helps clear up congestion. Chicken broth may also contain some enzymes that may have an anti-microbial effect. It is necessary for everyone to try healing with chicken soup recipe to banish your cold.

The cure eczema all you need to do is add a sprinkle of baking soda or even some uncooked oats to warm bath for skin-soothing effect. If that area becomes infected, then your doctor may recommend adding up a capful of bleach to your bath to get some relief.

The reason to this is that bleach kills any skin-irritating bacteria. You should make sure that you spend only five to 10 minutes in the tub and don't submerge your head in it. The emergency case that may require you to call your doctor is if you are too itchy to sleep, and you suspect that your skin is infected or your condition doesn't improve within a few days of treatment.

Chapter 1 – Getting Started

Every new thing you learn needs the proper tools to do it right. Don't worry. When making home remedies, it is best to avoid contamination as much as possible, but it won't require you turning your kitchen into a laboratory, and most of the things on the following list are probably already in your home:

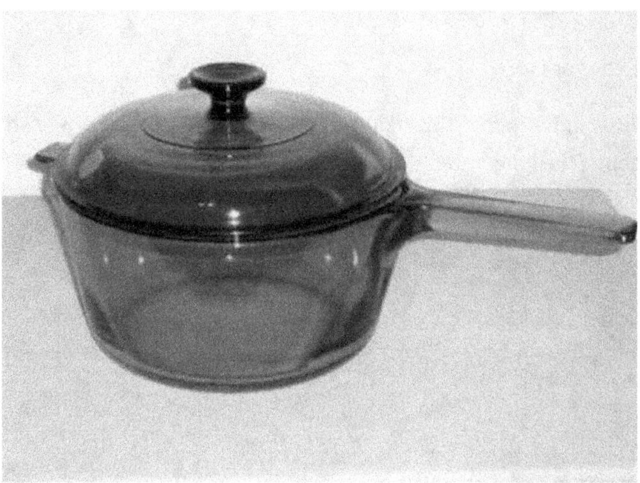

- Glass or porcelain pot or tea pot

    o Water can leach the properties of the metals it is boiled in. This can make the remedy have an unintended taste or not work as well.

    o Vision cookware is best, but you can still find porcelain tea pots on sale in department stores, if you don't already have the pots.

- Wooden spoons and ladles

- Coffee filters or cheesecloth

  - Some remedies require you to strain the herbs from the tea. These are two highly recommended ways of doing it.

- Porcelain or glass cups

  - This is for steeping teas.

- Dark glass bottles or jars

  - The less light going through the glass when storing oils and ointments, the longer those remedies last.

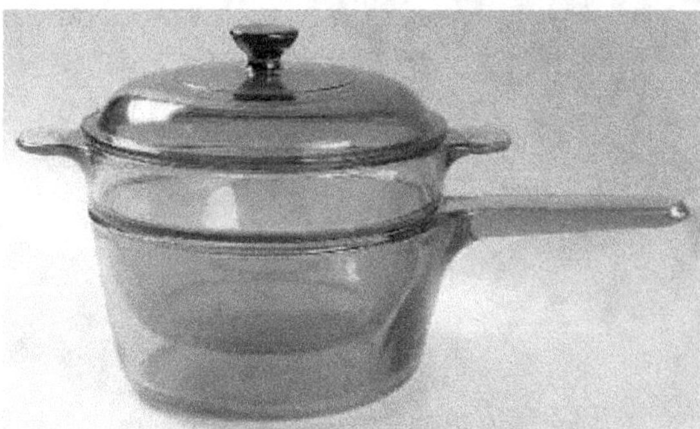

- Double boiler or Bain Marie

  - Some remedies will call for you to gently heat ingredients without them touching water. Again, please use either glass or porcelain.

- Porcelain or glass baking pan

- Crock pot

- o This is for making your herbal oils quicker than the conventional way.

- Candle Warmer

  - o If you don't have an essential oil diffuser, this is the next best thing. You can place the undiluted essential oils directly on the warmer.

Here are a few things you may not have thought of that are already in your kitchen:

- Coffee grinds

  - o These are perfect for facial masks and scrubs.

- Brown Sugar

  - o For sugar scrubs

- Baking soda

  - o For bath salts

- Sea salt

  - o For salt scrubs and bath salts

- Epsom Salts

  - o For mineral baths

- Borax

  - o This is a natural mineral that boosts that action of mineral bath salts.

- Whole Oats

  o Ground and added in place of salt, it makes for a soothing mineral bath.

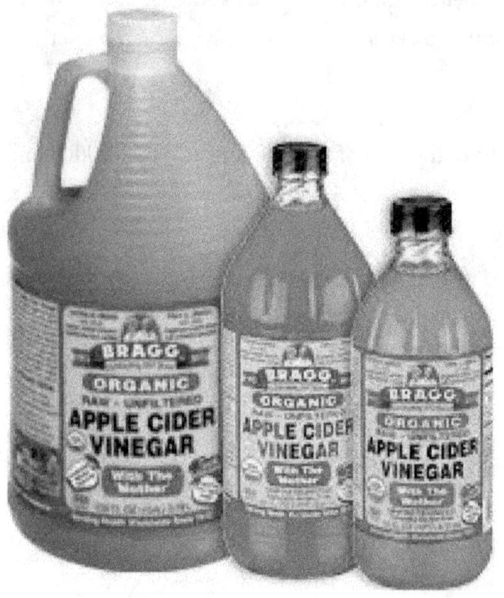

- Vinegar

  o Apple Cider Vinegar with the mother.

  o This is wonderful when mixed with a tea for cleansing the skin, and removing build-up from hair products.

- Olive Oil

  o Great for herbal oils

- Coconut Oil

    o Just like Olive oil, but it has more healing properties and you can even make it into ointments.

- Eggs

    o Good for conditioning hair.

    o Good for the skin as well.

As you can see, there are a lot of things you already have you can use to make remedies without breaking the bank. I will probably mention more that are not the list above in the recipes as we go on.

Chapter 2 –Spice Rack

You use it every day to add flair and flavor to your dishes. A little oregano here and a pinch of basil there, and you can even turn left-overs into a whole new dish, but did you know many of the herbs you cook with can also help heal you as well?

Allspice

This wonderful little herb who lends its flavor to many island dishes, also helps in cases of indigestion, intestinal cramping, and eve help relieve the swelling and of swollen joints from arthritis. It can be made into a tea, into an oil and even a bath.

Basil

This herb, which is in many households, is a champ when it comes to remedies which are home-made. It helps to tame gas, soothes nerves, calms nausea, can be used as an antihistamine, and is a good disinfectant. You can make it into a tea or oil.

Cinnamon

Cinnamon is used in confections and island dishes. The essential oil of this herb is used to calm the nerves and a nervous stomach. The powdered cinnamon is no different. It also provides natural caffeine, just a little bit. This herb is great as an oil.

Cayenne

Famous for adding heat to chili, Cayenne is also helpful in cases of intestinal problems, indigestion, and can loosen up phlegm caused by congestion. great for poultices, capsules, and ointments.

Cloves

This is another good one for indigestion and nausea. The juice from a single clove can stop nausea and the convulsion related to it. Just chew it to get the juice and spit out the clove.

Garlic

This wonder herb is known to boost the immune system, help lower high blood pressure and cholesterol, and even help in cases of congestion. You can eat it straight, but it's better served as an oil.

Ginger

Chewing on this herb in its candied form can help allay motion sickness. It is also great for lessening the severity and duration of colds and flu. The fresh juice is good in poultices and teas.

Bay (laurel) Leaves

We add these to stews and sometimes even chili, but did you know it can help heal a sprain, earaches, and even removes blockages that cause infections? It's true!

Marjoram

Another favorite in Italian dishes, Marjoram also helps to speed the healing in cases of sprains and can also heal bruises. Good in rubs and soaks.

Parsley

Yes, the green leafy spring on expensive restaurant plates is there for a reason. It helps to combat heartburn, gas, and bad breath. It can also help break-up kidney stones and treat insect bites. You can apply the juice by crushing the herb.

Pepper, Black

Usually paired with salt in restaurants, this herb, when made into a paste, can help soothe bronchitis and other chronic respiratory problems. You can put this in ointments and oils.

Onion

Though not an herb per se, can help in cases of water retention, earaches, coughs and colds. Make into an oil.

Rosemary

The herb that makes chicken sing and soups taste wonderful helps treat headaches, nervous tension, a nervous stomach, cleanse the face, and can even help to stimulate hair growth. Great in teas, oils, and soaks.

Sage

This is an herb no one that makes home remedies is caught without. It has antiseptic properties, anti-inflammation properties, can draw out toxins from bug bites, and even help to treat abscesses in the mouth. It's also helpful in healing ulcers. It's great in washes, teas, and ointments.

Thyme

This Italian herb is also known for helping in cases of sinus problems. It helps to break up impacted mucous. You can use it like Sage.

It's a long list, but a very helpful one when you're looking for something to make and have handy in case something happens or someone gets sick.

Herbs and Essential Oils you can add to it.

This list will cover essential oils and herbs you can find in health food and herb shops that are affordable. Adding these to your home remedy list will have you prepared for anything.

Aloe

The all-natural gel or juice is the best. Most of the aloes you get in bottles during the summer have been diluted with alcohol. You can use this as a base for many spot treatments.

Calendula Petals

Most commonly known as Marigold, this herb can speed clotting and is a strong antiviral in cases of colds and flu.

Chamomile

This herb can be found in the tea section of any grocery store. You can combine it with some of the cooking herbs above for skin problems and soothing the stomach.

Echinacea

Many places sell this as a tea as well, which comes in handy if you're making poultices or compresses. It boosts the immune system and speeds the healing of cuts, scrapes, and bruises.

Feverfew

Coupled with Rosemary, it's a powerful punch for treating headaches, migraines, and cluster headaches. This herb alone can do it, but sometimes even the best herb for the job can use a helping hand.

Green Tea

Though many don't consider this tea an herb, it actually is. It is packed with antioxidants and antivirals to help you take care of mouth problems and kick colds.

White Oak Bark

This one can be found in health food stores, herb shops and online. As a powder, you can make into a poultice for bug bites. It draws out the toxins.

Lavender Essential oil

This versatile essential oil can help in first aid heal burns and sooth itching. It also helps to reduce inflammation.

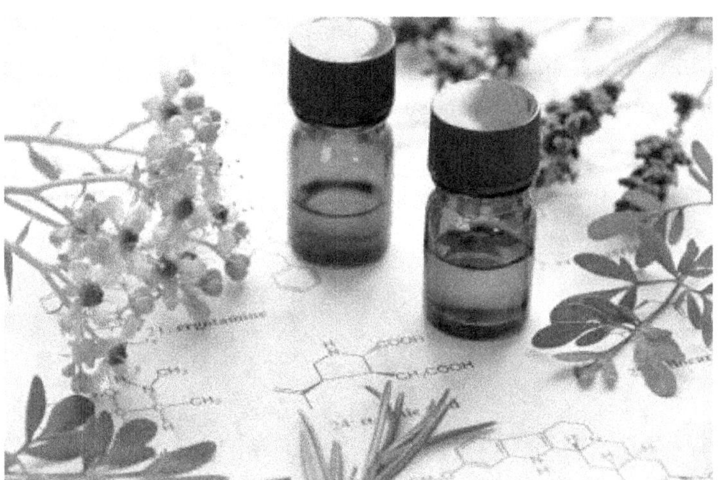

Lemon Essential oil
This oil can kill germs and when used with Peppermint, Echinacea, and Sage, it can help to speed the healing of cuts, scrapes and bruises.

Peppermint Essential oil
This oil not only smells heavenly, but can be used in a pinch, mixed with a lotion as a penetrating chest rub or added to a poultice to help open up a congested chest. You can also add it to water to make a disinfectant and even deter fleas.

Tea Tree Essential oil

This essential oil is a great germ fighter. You can add it to water for a spot disinfectant or even put a few drops on a candle warmer to kill airborne germs.

There are a lot more herbs you can get to supplement this list, but this is a list of the most readily available and most affordable. Some herbs and essential oils can cost upwards of $20.00 or more for the smallest of bottles.

Chapter 3 – Useful Tips

When taking herbal supplements and remedies on a regular basis, you need to take heed about possible interactions that may happen if you are on prescription medications. These can range from mildly irritating to possible life-threatening.

Blood thinners and Blood pressure medications
There are some herbs that can thin the blood, lower, and even raise blood pressure. If you are taking any of these types of prescription medicine, avoid these types of herbs.

If you are on high blood pressure medications, avoid using Rosemary in therapeutic does as it may cause a spike in blood pressure, counteracting the medication.

Antidepressants
If you are on antidepressants, avoid taking herbals that do the same thing. This will cause euphoria and can lead to injury down the road.

Diabetes
There are herbs out there that can raise or lower your blood sugar. Some of these, like Stevia and Nopal, can be fine when you monitor your blood sugar and adjust accordingly, but do so cautiously. Golden Seal, an immune booster, can drastically lower blood sugar and should be avoided by people with blood sugar problems.

Auto-immune diseases

We all want to feel better, but if you are suffering from an auto-immune disease, consult your doctor and a naturopath to see if taking herbs can be beneficial and which ones to avoid so you don't block the action of existing treatments.

You and your doctor

If you are going in for tests and you're taking herbal supplements, you may have to stop taking those as well. Many herbs, taken in either maintenance or therapeutic does, can skew test results. Let your doctor know what you are taking.

Chapter 4 Recipes: Part 1

Aloe Vera:

Aloe Vera is considered to be a very useful medicinal herb. It is widely known as skin friendly and hair friendly herb. It is one of the safe herbs which do not require any processing before its use. These can be easily cultivated in the garden and the pot. These plants are easily grown in hot climates and can resist harsh environment.

This plant is used for dry, inflamed or abraded skin. It is also used for minor cuts and sunburns. It also possesses antibacterial and anti-inflammatory effects. It is also edible and can be utilized for gastrointestinal ailments like constipation, irritable bowel syndrome and ulcerative colitis, etc.

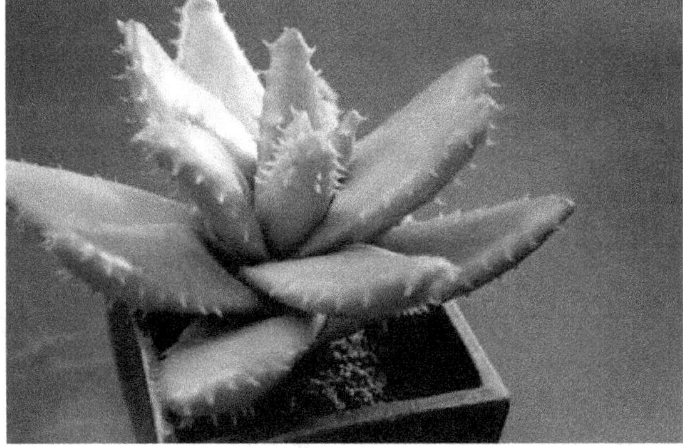

Garlic

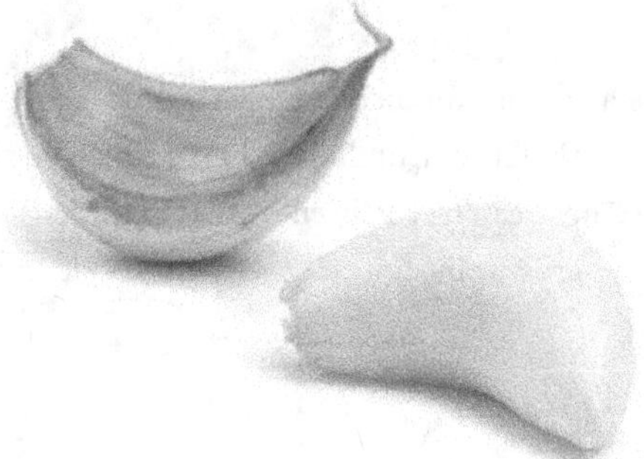

Garlic is available in every kitchen, and it is excellent home remedies to treat a lot of different bacterial and fungal infection. I would also like to suggest that it is a good way to treat bacterial infection by eating at least 4 to 5 cloves of garlic per day.

Moreover, garlic is also considered good for your digestive system. There are multiple yet different ways for you to consume the intake of garlic. You can either chew it or even swallow it. Another way is eating garlic in the form of pharmaceutical capsules.

However, there may be very less and ineffective than directly chewing garlic. Moreover, garlic tea is also another option and recommendation as all the herbal remedy on how to treat and cure your bacterial infection. You would want to add some cloves in the boiling water and steep them some of a few minutes before they are sipping the garlic tea.

Garlic can also be consumed in many ways. The best way is, however, to chew garlic and swallow them raw.

Capsules are widely available as well, even though they might not be as effective. Garlic tea can also help to prepared from boiling some few cloves of garlic and steeping it for at least ten minutes.

Peppermint:

It is a herb that is available in every household and is widely used. It is also part of products manufactured for mouth freshener, dental hygiene, candies and soothing balms. It is used as a medicinal herb since very ancient time. Tea made up of peppermint can relieve stomach upsets and relieve pain and discomfort due to gas. Sniffing of its leaves can also be sooth nausea and vomiting. It has an ingredient called menthol that gives a cooling effect to the skin. It can relieve itching and burning conditions of the skin. It can also relieve muscle cramps and headache because of its analgesic effects.

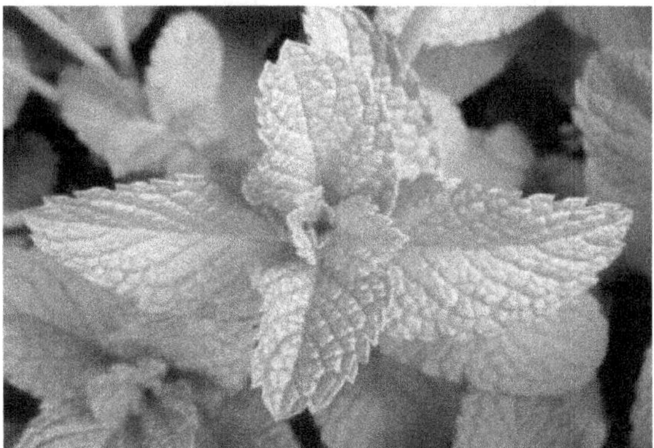

Valerian

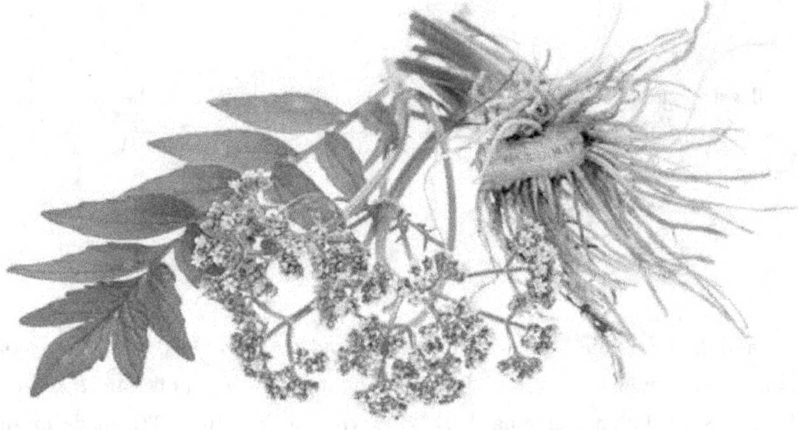

Valerian is also another very popular nighttime home remedies to deal with your anxiety. It contains some elements of mild tranquilizing properties that will almost guarantee you and will get you a good night sleep. However, without all dreaded and the weird hangover feeling early in the morning that you may sometimes have to get with some other pharmaceuticals.

Thyme:

It is an aromatic herb that can be easily cultivated in a sunny climate. It can also bear the harsh climate of an area. It contains a volatile oil called thymol that is liberated even upon slight touch. Thymol is an alcohol which is an antiseptic. It is used in the treatment of tonsillitis and laryngitis. It can be used for getting rid of bad smell from the mouth by doing gargle with its water. Nervous exhaustion can be relieved by sniffing its leaves. It is widely used in the treatment of respiratory infections bronchitis, chest congestion, asthma, and whooping cough.

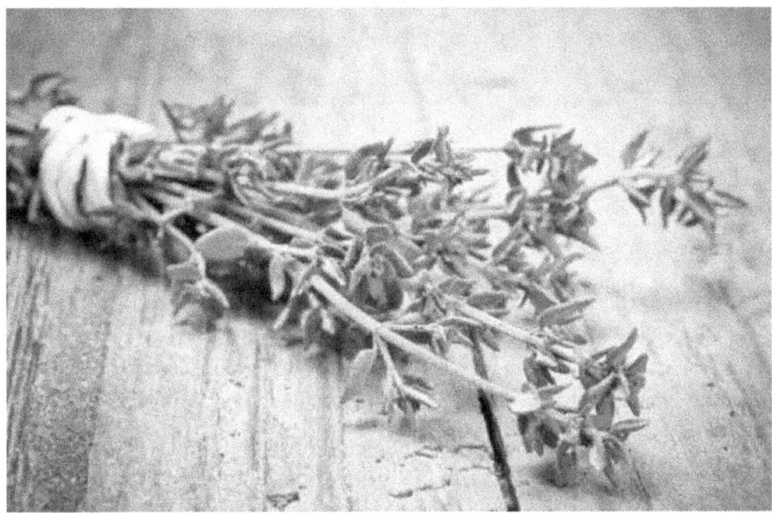

Passionflower

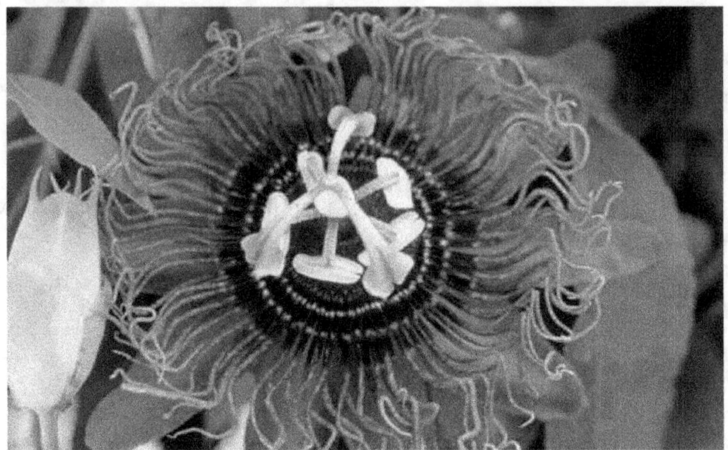

Passionflower is also referred to as folk for a natural remedy and anxiety, insomnia and panic attacks. Passionflower has been shown in many studies to treat anxiety is a very remarkably well.

One study has found it has to be as effective as benzodiazepine drugs, but the only difference is without the drowsiness. Passionflower may also help you to feel an emotionally balanced and exceptionally beneficial way.

Nonetheless, if you suffer from exaggerated emotions then this is by far one of the most efficient home remedies to deal with anxiety, and it needs to be part of your daily regimen.

Rosemary:

Rosemary is more like a woody plant that is also used for medicinal purposes. It is used for the treatment of general ailments rather than the specific ones. It contains carsonic acid nullify the effects of beta-amyloid peptide that results in neurodegeneration and brain damage. These peptides are the cause of Alzheimer's disease. Its oil can enhance cognitive functions and prevent aging of the brain.

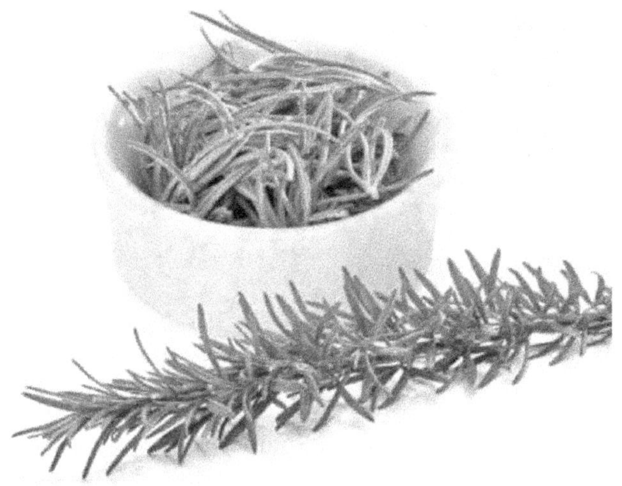

Lemon Balm

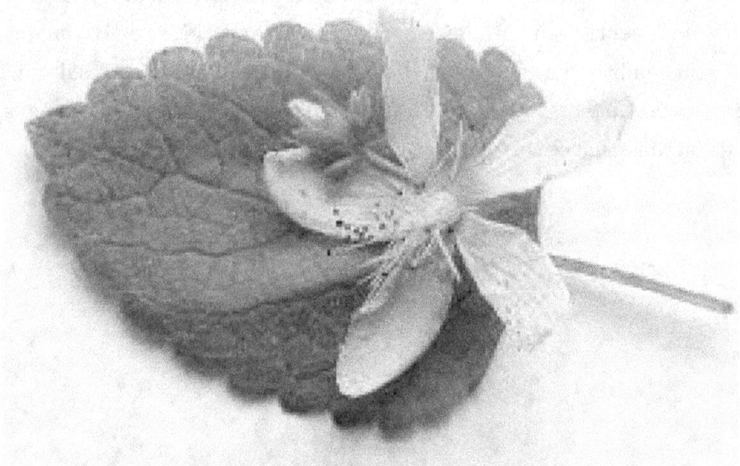

Lemon Balm also is known as 'Melissa officinalis' which is one herbal supplement and tea to treat anxiety and calm your nerves. Some studies suggested that the use of lemon balm can decrease insomnia, anxiety, hyper excitation and fatigue.

A lemon balm extract which should be taken 300mg at breakfast and 300mg at dinner too which may help reduced insomnia mainly due to a decrease in nervousness and also to decreased agitation, guilt, hyperexcitation and fatigue too.

Chamomile

This herb is the core for the treatment of chest problems. There are many types of chamomile, but one with medicinal use is the Roman chamomile. The Roman chamomile is just like German chamomile in loose, so the scientific names are necessary for its identification. It's tea can be used for relaxation of mind or treatment of abdominal cramps.

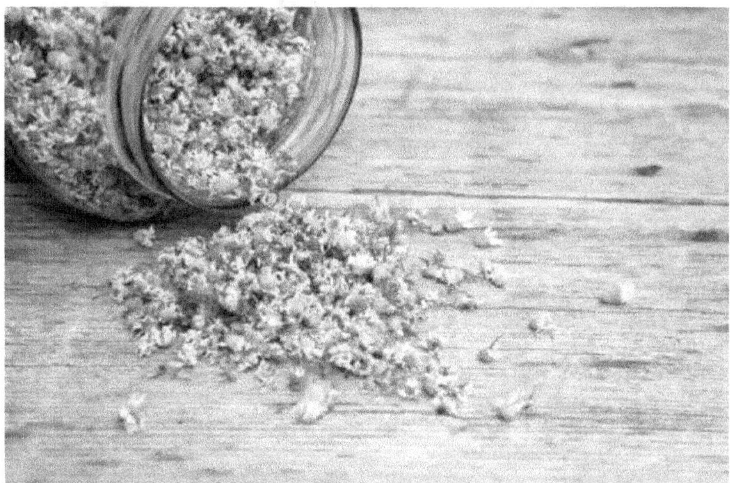

This is the part of the book you've been waiting for, but you're going to need to learn a few terms and preparations first. So, let's get that list out of the way.

California poppy

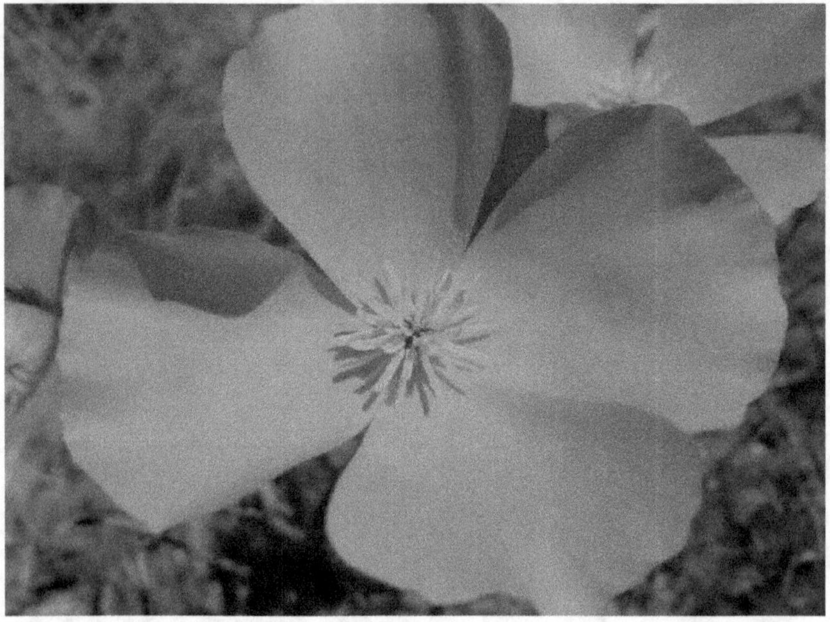

California poppy also called Eschscholtzia californica, which is a tension-relieving, anti-anxiety, sedative, and antispasmodic herb. California poppy also helps with sleeplessness and quells a headache as well as muscular spasm from stress. Some gentle and non-addictive actions are much safer for children and the elderly.

Pot marigold:

These are the flowers with yellow or orange petals. They can be grown in some climates disregarding pH and soil fertility.

This flower has antiseptic properties. It can be used for any ailment related to skin. It is the active ingredient of almost every skin ointment, and it can be utilized for any skin disease. It also reduces inflammation and stops bleeding.

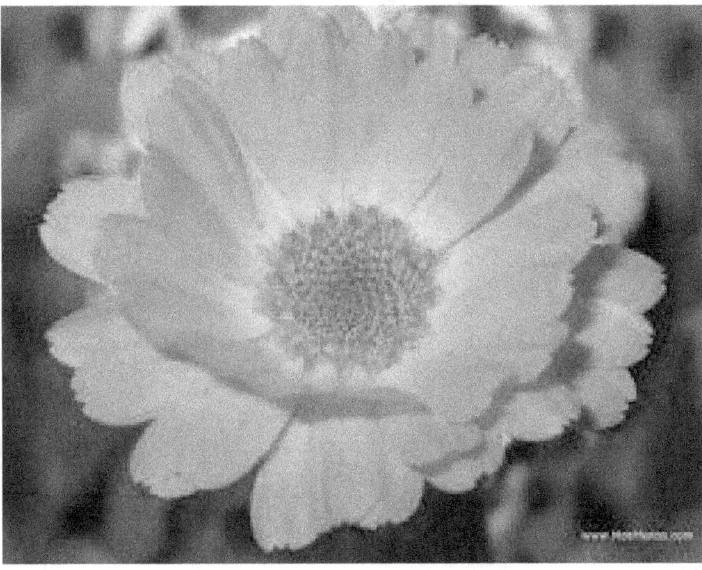

Sage (Salvia officinalis):

It is used as a medicinal plant for a long time. It is also used for cooking. It improves appetite and prevents flatulence. This plant has a regulatory effect on hormone regulation in human. It can be utilized for treatment. It also relieves respiratory symptoms. It has neuroprotective effects and be used for the treatment of dementia, Alzheimer's, etc. it also treats diaphoresis.

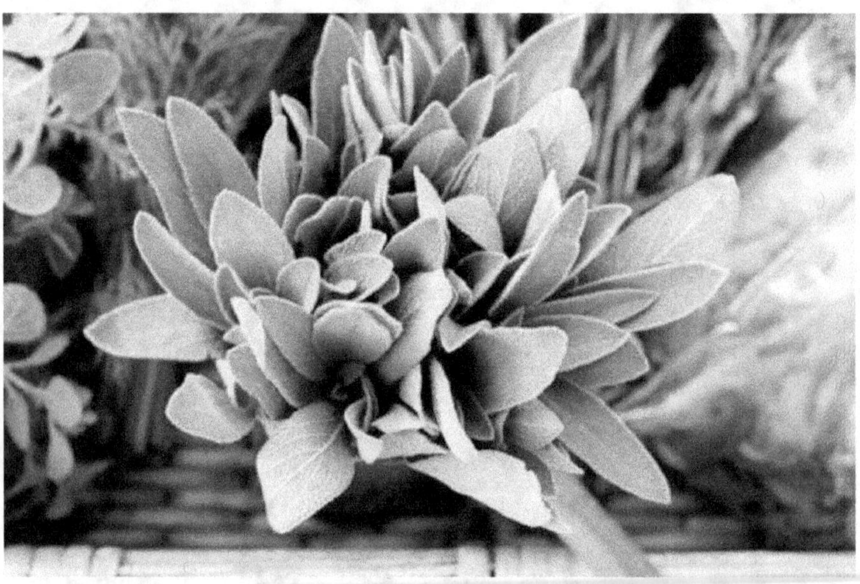

Wild Lettuce

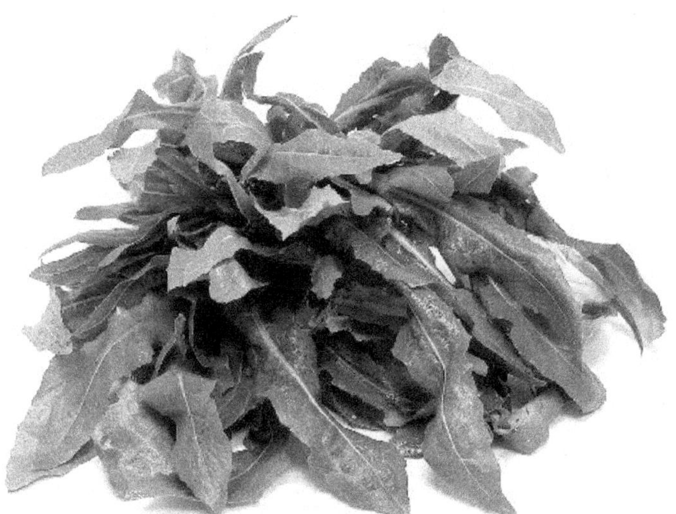

Wild Lettuce is of the species of lactic vireos, which is a mild tranquilizer that may be used for calming a nervous or overactive nervous system. It is very suitable for anxious children or even adolescents. It majorly helps with insomnia. It is also a general pain reliever and antispasmodic that can primarily be used for short coughs.

Lavender (Lavandula angustifolia)

This herb has its medicinal property and is also used as a herb. It is widely used for ornamental purposes as well. It is useful in the treatment of a headache and depression. It can also be used for the treatment of insomnia. It also has antiseptic and anti bacterial properties.

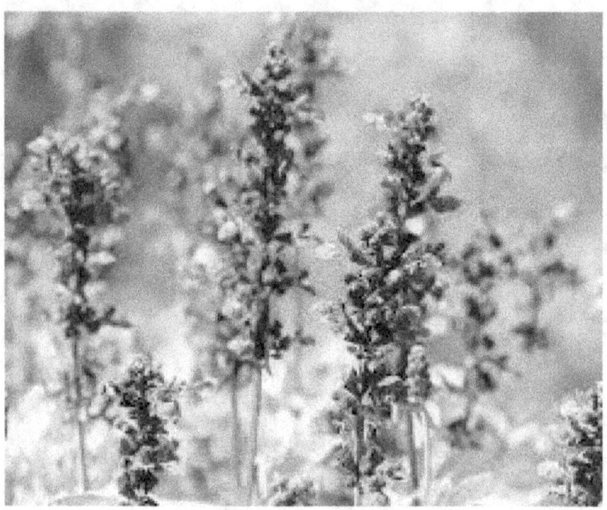

Echinacea (E. purpurea / E. Angustifolia):

It is hail from North America. These are grown in sunny weather. It increases the power of the immune system and helps in fighting with bacterial and viral infections. They are extensively used for the treatment of flu, cold, wounds, insect bites, burns, and snake bites.

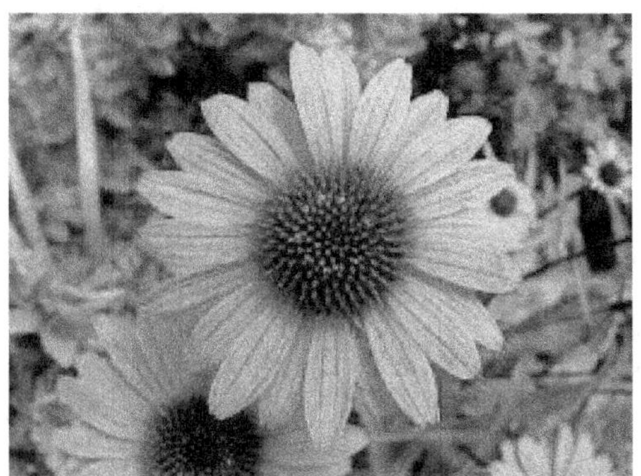

Comfrey (Symphytum officinale)

These are another medicinal plant that is widely used for the treatment of ligament injuries and broken bones. Because of these properties they are also known as boneset and knit bone. They are also used for the treatment of arthritic pain, varicose vein ulcers, dysmenorrhea, increased menstrual flow, gastrointestinal problem, stomach ulcers, and sore throat and gum diseases. However, now a day's only topical application is recommended.

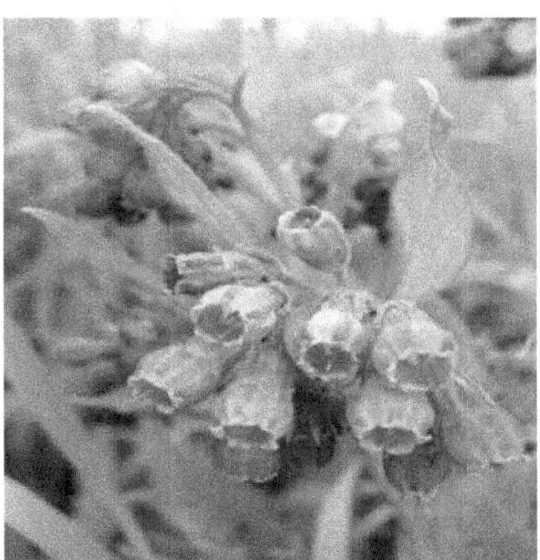

Broadleaf plantain (Plantago major)

This plant is considered to be a weed. It also carries certain antimicrobial, anti-inflammatory and wound-healing properties. Its leaves are also used for the treatment of wounds, insect bites and skin sores for the relief of pain and to promote healing. It is also used for the treatment of diarrhea and gout.

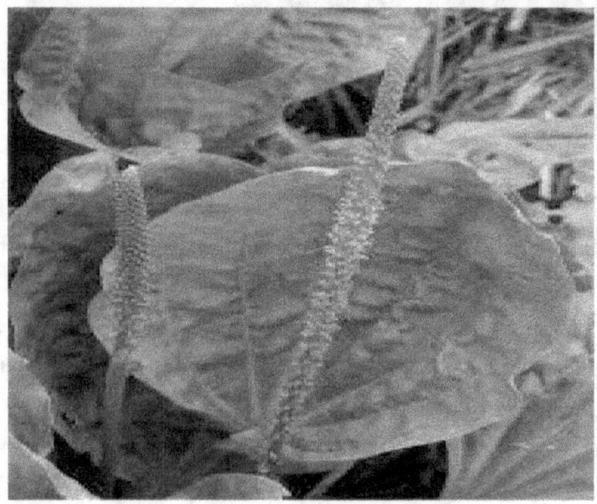

Chapter 5 Recipes: Part 2

Compress

This can made from teas and essential oils. This is a bowl of warm to hot water with medicinal properties which can be placed, via a clean damp towel, on the affected area. It is switched out when the towel gets cool.

Treatment of Itching with Clay

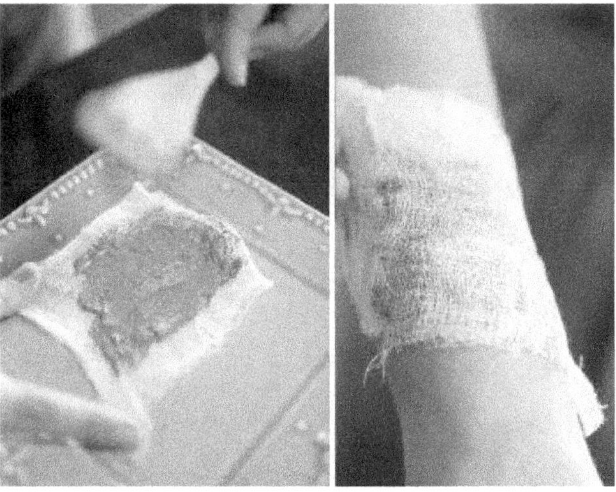

Clay is good for the treatment of itching, acne and various other issues related to your skin. If you want to use clay, mix one cup clay in a bowl and mix it with a small quantity of filtered water to make a creamy paste. Dab your itchy areas with this clay paste and let it dry.

Clay Pack

Spread your clay paste on one piece of clean fabric (cotton, muslin, wool and flannel). Put this clay cloth on irritated area so that the clay should directly touch your skin. A bandage wrap or tape can be used to fix this clay patch on your skin for almost four hours.

Decoction

This is a teas made from boiling roots, stems, and bark. These ingredients take longer to extract the medicinal properties out of them. They need 20 minutes on a low boil. These can store in a refrigerator for about a week.

Oat meal paste:

Oat meal has cleansing property. This cleansing property helps to remove scars of the skin.

Ingredients:

Oat meal

Water

Procedure:

Take a small amount of water in a blender. Ass some amount of water into it. Turn on the blender and make a thick paste. Apply this paste as a mask over your face. Allow it dry for at least 15 minutes or more. Rinse it off with Luke warm water. Dry your face with a towel. Repeat this procedure twice a week. This will reduce acne marks from your face.

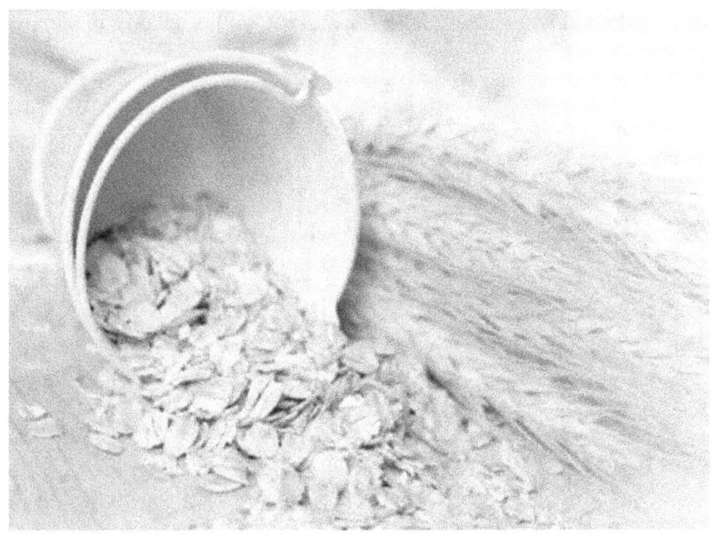

Herbal Baths

This is the practice of taking four ounces of herbs and sewing, or placing them, into a pillow case or other bag that allow the water to flow into it. You place it in a tub of warm to hot running water and soak up the medicine. These are one-shot.

Herbal oil

You can make this two ways:

1. Adding an ounce of dried herbs to a pint of oil in a glass jar and leaving it for three weeks in a warm place.

2. Adding an ounce of dried herbs to a pint of oil in a crock pot on low overnight.

I personally use the second method. Crock pots get just hot enough to help release the heating properties of the herbs without frying the plant material.

Depending on the oil you use and how you store it, an herbal oil can last up to six months in a cool dry place.

Apple Cider and Clay Recipe

Apple cider can be a good choice to relieve itching with its anti-bacterial and anti-fungal properties. You can use this treatment for dandruff and sunburns. You can directly apply apple vinegar on your skin by putting some drops on washcloth or cotton ball.

If you want to make a clay pack with vinegar, you can substitute water with apple vinegar and make a smooth mixture. You can mix well until you get desired consistency. Apply this paste on a bandage and put clay area on your skin for almost four hours. You can replicate this treatment twice a week.

Infusion

This is a tea made from the leaves and flowers of the herbs. Traditionally, you make it buy running a pint of water through herbs placed on a strainer, but for book purposes, you can make them buy adding water to a cup or bowl which has the herbs already in them. These take 10 minutes to steep to get the most benefit from the medicinal properties. These last about as long as decoctions.

Lavender flower:

Lavender has already been used for many ailments. Its anti-septic and anti-bacterial properties allow it to be used for particular skin problems.

Ingredients:
Lavender flower

Water

Cotton pad

Procedure:

Take a small amount of water in a pan. Add some flowers of lavender into it. Boil this water. Take it out in a bowl. Let it cool. Apply this tonic to the damaged skin or acne with the help of cotton pad or directly. You can also save this water in a bottle and save it for later use.

Lemon paste:

Lemon is regarded one of the best ingredients for the treatment of skin problems. Citric acid present in lemon is used for removing dead cells. Vitamin C is an anti-oxidant present in lemon which helps to reduce dark spots on the skin. It also has bleaching puppetries which enhance complexion of the skin.

Ingredients:

Lemon juice

Sugar

Procedure:

Mix lemon juice with some sugar but do not dissolve the sugar. Apply this mixture on the face, hand, and neck. Rub this in a circular motion with light hands for five minutes. Leave it for 10 to 15 minutes. Wash your face with Luke warm water. This will provide you an instant glow to your face.

Massage oils

This is an oil to which herbs or essential oils or both have been added. You can use this to sooth tight muscles, treat bruises, and even soften skin, depending on the ingredients. These can last about as long as herbal oils.

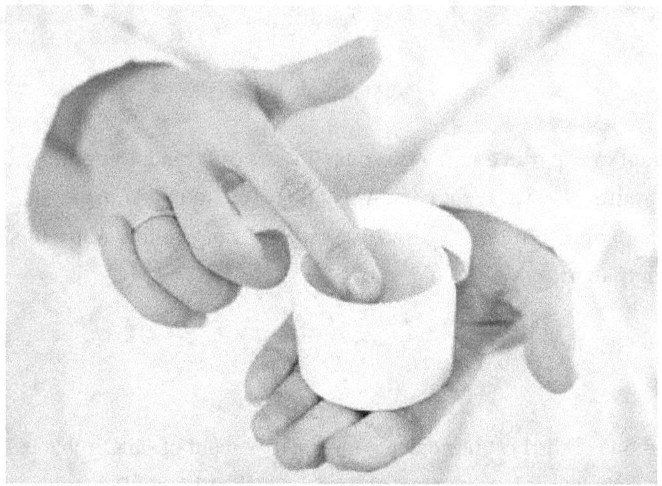

Mineral Baths

This is a combination of Borax, Sea Salt, Epsom Salt, and Baking Soda. You can add herbs and essential oils to the mix to speed healing, detox your body, or just relax. If you have high blood pressure, it is recommended you substitute the salts for ground oatmeal. If you make a large batch, it can store up to six months before the potency starts to wane.

Cucumber paste:

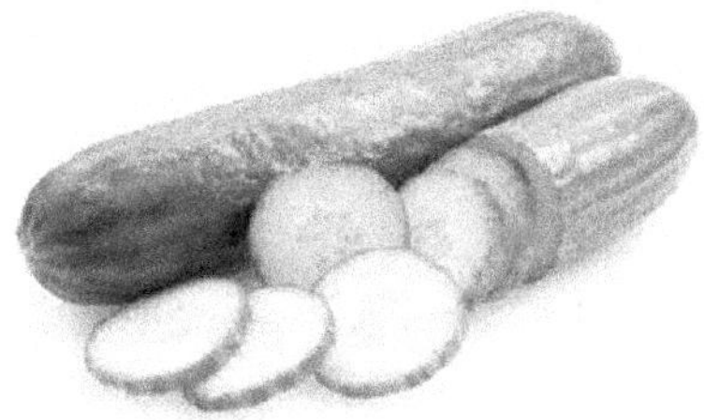

Cucumber has a lot of water content and minerals. They allow you to repair damaged skin, removing dead cells and add a fresh glow.

Ingredients:

Cucumber juice

Lemon juice

Procedure:

Take one tablespoon of cucumber juice and one tablespoon of lemon juice. Mix them together. Apply this onto the face and leave it until dry. Wash your face with Luke warm water and dry it with the towel. Follow this remedy daily until the situation wards off.

Procedure to Use

You can break off leaves from its plant and cut to open lengthwise from the bottom and top with the help of a knife. Scoop all gooey gel out and carefully rub it on your affected skin and leave it for almost 15 minutes. You can do it on a regular basis until cured. Left over gel can be secured in one airtight container for almost one week.

The rheumatoid arthritis is related to the immune system, and become the reason of inflammation of joints and tissues. The immune system can disturb your overall healthy tissues and organs. You can apply the aloe vera gel to your joint to treat arthritis:

- If you want to get the best results, directly take the plants. It will help you to relieve pain and swelling linked with the rheumatoid arthritis. Cut the leaf from an aloe vera plant with the help of a sharp scissor, and peel its outer leaf to get the gel. You can use your fingers to get the gel out from the plant. Spread the gel on the affected parts just like a lotion, and massage these parts.

- You can also drink the aloe vera juice for the treatment of arthritis. Start your treatment with the small dose that can be 2 to 3 ounces once in a day. You can increase this quantity up to 3 times per day. It will help you to take care of the tenderness in your body, as well as the digestive system.

- You can use aloe vera treatment with other remedies as well because the aloe vera is not only sufficient to treat the rheumatoid arthritis.

Ointments

These can be tricky to make, but they can last a while. You start by warming a base oil and adding the herbs. You then strain out the herbs and add the oil to a double boiler. You then add beeswax to the oil. If you are adding essential oils to this, it is recommended you wait unit the mixture is Luke warm.

Baking Soda

The baking soad always proves good to treat rashes of your skin. It has ability to relieve itching and the inflammation that is associated with rashes.

Procedure to Use Baking Soda

To work with baking soda, you should take one part of baking soda and mix it with three parts of water. Apply this mixture on particular area of your skin and wait for five minutes before washing your face. You can practice this almost twice in one day and see the improvement.

It is easy to mix some baking soda and coconut oil to make a smooth paste and apply this paste on your rashes. Leave this paste on your skin for almost five minutes and wash your wash. Replicate this procedure twice a day and see improvements.

Poultice

A poultice is a thick paste made of herbs, essential oils, and water. This can be applied directly to wounds and bruises to pull out infections and speed healing. These are generally one-shot as you make them when you need them.

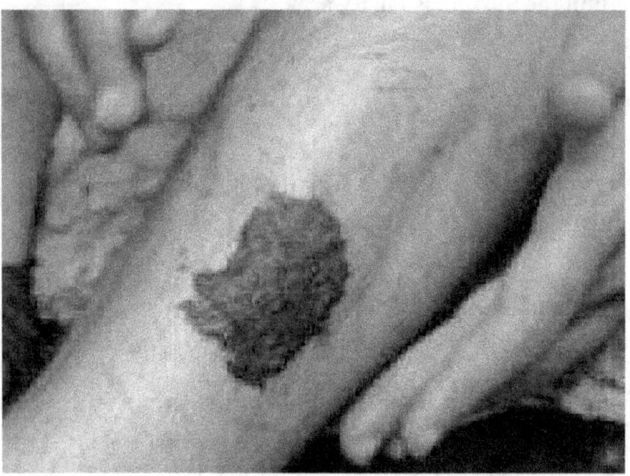

Syrups

These are cough syrups you can make at home with water, herbs, and honey. It takes two ounces of the herb, one quart of water, and two ounces of honey. These can last up to a week in the refrigerator.

Turmeric paste:

Turmeric has anti-septic, and skin is glowing agents. It can be used to treat scars on the skin. It is also helpful for treatment of allergic, inflammatory and infectious skin diseases.

Ingredients:

Turmeric powder

Pineapple juice

Take a small amount of turmeric powder and mix it with pineapple juice. Make a paste out of it. Apply this paste on the face, hands, and neck. Leave this paste on the skin until it is dried. Once it is dried, wash it with Luke warm water. Follow this remedy for twice or thrice a week. This will reduce inflammation and allergy of the skin. This also allows brightening your skin.

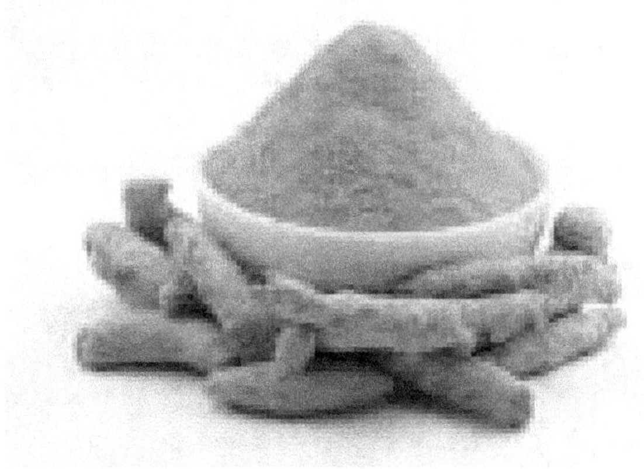

Wound wash

Just as it sounds, you mix tea and essential oils in a squeeze bottle and squirt it in the scrape or cut to wash out any dirt particles and clean the wound. This is a quick way to clean and disinfect a cut or scrape. These are immediate use.

Valerian Root

Valerian is a herb, and its roots are used to make medicine for sleep disorders. It is a common herb used with the combination of hops and lemon balms. The valerian root can cause drowsiness and is ideal for those suffering from the insomnia.

If you are using sleeping pills, then you are advised to treat it with valerian root. There are some scientific evidences that the valerian works for the treatment of sleep disorders. It can also help you to treat the conditions connected with the anxiety and psychological stress that may be asthma, excitants, migraine, headache, upset stomach, etc. It can also be used for the treatment of depression, epilepsy, mild tremors and chronic fatigue.

The women suffering from the menstrual cramps and symptoms of menopause, they can use this herb for their treatment. The extracts and oil of the valerian root are used to flavor different food items and beverages.

How does it work?

The valerian works like a tranquilizer on your brain and nervous system. Its continuous use will help you to get rid of sleeping pills. It will improve your sleep quality, and bring lots of other benefits with it.

Side Effects

The Valerian is quite safe to use for the people using it for the medicinal purpose. You can use it for almost 4 to 8 weeks on a constant basis for desired results. There are different side effects of valerian noticed by some people are headache, excitability, and uneasiness.

Some people may have sluggish feelings after having it in the night, but these side effects will be temporary. It will be good to gradually reduce the use of valerian before quitting it completely.

Interactions of Valerian

- If you are taking valerian, then you have to avoid the use of alcohol because alcohol can be the reason of drowsiness and tiredness.

- The alprazolam can also interact with the valerian because taking both of them at the same time can increase its side effects.

- Benzodiazepine is a sedative medicine and it can strongly interact with valerian causing sleepiness. There is no need to take any sleeping pill and valerian at the same time.

Accurate Dosage of Valerian

- If you are suffering from insomnia, then you can take valerian by mouth in the following ways:
- 400 to 900 mg valerian should be extracted for two hours of your sleep time, and you can take it for almost 28 days.
- The 120 mg valerian can be combined with 80 mg lemon balm to take for almost 30 days. Its regular dosage will be 3 times a day.
- You can take the combination of 187 mg valerian extract and make a tablet of 41.9 mg to take almost 2 tablets of the similar quantity at the bedtime for almost 28 days.

Now we're ready to get to it. These recipes will start with the top of the body and their way down.

Headache Remedies
Rosemary and Thyme Sinus Pack
1 tbsp ground whole oats

1 tsp Rosemary leaves

1 tsp Thyme leaves

1/4 boiled water

5 Drops Peppermint essential oil

2 Drops of Lavender essential oi

2 Drops of Lemon essential oil

- Add the Rosemary and Thyme to the boiled water.

- Cover and let steep for ten minutes

- Add just enough of the strong infusion to make a paste.

- Add the essential oils and mix well.

- Place the poultice around the eyes, being careful not get any in the eyes.

- Leave on for twenty minutes before washing off.

Headache Tea

1 tsp Feverfew

1/2 tsp Rosemary

1 Drop Peppermint essential oil

- Boil one cup of water, about 6 ounces.

- Add the water the herbs and let steep for ten minutes.

- Strain out the herbs, add the peppermint, and a little honey.

Broad leaf plantain tea:

Broad leaf plantain can be used for the treatment of diarrhea and gout. Aucubin in broad leaf plantain increase secretion of uric acid from the kidney thus, helping relief of symptoms of gout.

Ingredients:

Broad leaf plantain

Water

Procedure;

Take some amount of water in a pot. Add leaves of broad leaf plant into it. Boil it to make a tea. Take it out in a cup and drink it. It will relieve diarrhea and kidney stone formation. Its leaves can be chewed as it is for relieving of these diseases.

Headache Herbal oil

1/2 Ounce of Feverfew

1/2 Ounce of Rosemary

1 pint of Olive oil

1/2 tbsp of peppermint

- Place the herbs in a crock pot.

- Add the oil

- Let run on low overnight.

- Add the essential oil.

- Mix well.

- Apply to temples, base of the neck, and the bridge of your nose.

Chamomile

Chamomile was a traditional medicine used thousands of years ago for the treatment of anxiety and upset stomach. It is still in use because of its amazing properties because it is considered as a safe plant and used to treat stomach ailments and sleeplessness.

The herb is used with the combination of other plants to get lots of health benefits. If you are suffering from heartburn, upset stomach, nausea, and queasiness, then you can use chamomile. It also proves helpful for the sore mouth and cancer. If you have any skin irritation, the chamomile can help you to heal your wounds.

Dose of Chamomile

A standard dosage of the chamomile may vary between 400 milligrams and 1,600 milligrams in a day. You can take it in the form of a capsule, or prepare the tea to drink one to four cups a day. You can use flowers of chamomile to prepare the tea bags, and dip the tea bag in a cup of hot water and cover with a lid for almost 5 to 10 minutes. It is a safe drink for you, but you are advised to let it cool down before drinking it. You can add chamomile flavor for your food items and drinks.

Side Effects of Chamomile

Some experts suggested that the chamomile is quite safe to use, but its large doses can cause vomiting. It can also trigger some allergic reactions to the people suffering from relevant allergies with the plants of a daisy family.

- If you are using skin creams of chamomile, you should consider your typical allergic reactions because the chamomile can cause irritation to eyes and eczema.

- You are advised to consult your doctor before taking chamomile because it has a minute amount of coumarin that may affect the thinness of your blood. In some cases, the chamomile is taken before surgery to make your blood thinner, but don't forget to consider its interactions with the anesthetic drugs.

Interactions of Chamomile

- If you are taking any drug on a regular basis, such as aspirin, antiplatelet, NSAID painkillers, naproxen, ibuprofen and any other related drugs; you have to consult your doctor before taking chamomile supplements.
- The chamomile can interact with ginkgo Biloba, saw palmetto, valerian, and garlic. It is not advised to take it with any of these herbs.
- The chamomile is not good for pregnant and breastfeeding women. You have to take expert advice before giving it to infants and children.

Ginger tea with Turmeric

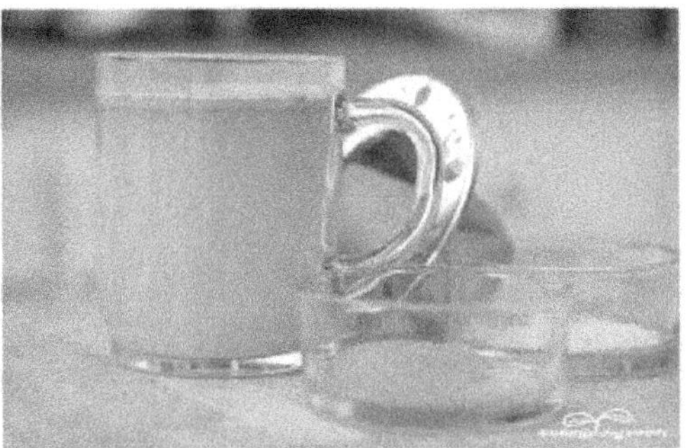

Turmeric is the herbal which we usually use in the food for the taste but it has a lot of benefits especially for the painful areas. They work as anti to the pains of osteoporosis and the rheumatoid. It has antioxidants which help you release the pain without causing any kind of inflammation. You can make it easily with these ingredients right at your home.

Ingredients:

- Water (2 cups)
- Ginger (grounded, about half teaspoon)
- Turmeric (grounded, about half teaspoon)
- Honey according to the taste

Directions:

Put about 2 cups of water into the put and let it boil. Then add the ginger and the turmeric powder in it and let it cook. Make sure that it is fully cooked because turmeric will be effective when it is fully cooked. When you are done, then pour it in the cup and add honey accordingly. You can make it and keep it stored to have it for more than once in the day.

Fevers

For a head cold

Compress

2 Tbsp Echinacea

1/2 tbsp Rosemary

1/2 tbsp Thyme

1/2 tbsp Feverfew

- Boil water and add the above ingredients.

- Strain out the herbs

- Damp a clean cloth

- Place on forehead

- change when the cloth is cool

- If needed, reheat the water.

Passionflower

The above part of the passionflower plant is used to make medicine for the sleep problems, anxiety, gastrointestinal ailments, nervousness and withdrawal symptoms of the narcotic drugs. It is equally beneficial for the asthma, hysteria, seizures, nervousness, irregular heartbeat and high blood pressure.

It can also be used to treat skin burns, pains and swelling. Its extracts are used in the food and beverages to flavor them. It can be used with the combination of other drugs to prop up tranquility and relaxation.

You can combine it with the hops, skullcap, kava, valerian and German chamomile. The chemicals found in the passionflower can make you calm and promote good sleep by relieving the effects of muscle spasm.

Side Effects of Passionflower

- The passion flower is found in the food and taken orally to treat insomnia. It should be taken in smaller amounts for the short period of time.
- The passionflower can cause confusion, giddiness, and irregular muscle functions. It may be the reason of inflamed blood vessels.
- You may feel nausea, vomiting, increase in the heart rate and irritations on the skin.
- Interactions of the Passionflower

The passionflower can interact with the narcotic medications because it can cause sleepiness with the use of sedative drugs. It should not be good to use with pentobarbital (Nembutal), Phenobarbital, secobarbital, clonazepam, lorazepam, zolpidem, and other drugs.

Dose of Passionflower

If you want to take passionflower by mouth, following are some dosage details for you:

- For the treatment of generalized anxiety disorder, you can take 45 drops of the passion flower liquid on a regular basis.
- A 90 mg tablet can also be used for the treatment of GAD.
- If you want to reduce the symptoms of narcotic withdrawal, then you can use 60 drops of the passionflower in a liquid with 0.8 mg of clonidine.

The Epsom Salt

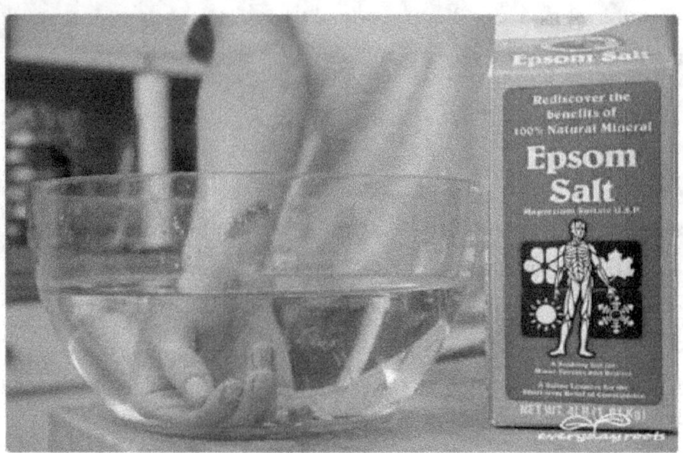

Epsom salt can help you release stress from your daily life routine. Even if you do not have any pain, you should try it once in a while and you will feel a lot better than before. If you want you can be consistent at it and you will see how it affects you with ease. It helps you release any joint pain whether it is your finger or your feet. Here is how you can make use of the Epsom Salt.

Ingredients

- Epson Salt (half cup)
- Bowl
- Water (Luke warm)

Directions:

Take the warm water in the bowl and add Epsom salt in it. Mix it well when you see it completely dissolved. Now you can soak your hands and feet in it and relax for as long as you want.

To get the full treatment, close your eyes and lay your back on the support. Forget everything for a while and you will see how easy you will be feeling once you are done. When you are done, then wash your feet and hand with plain water but make sure it should be warm too.

Parsley water:

Parsley water is a refreshing drink that can be taken after dinner. It can be used for the treatment of urinary tract infection. It also acts as a diuretic which discards off excess water from the body. Diuretic also decreases blood pressure. Because of this discarding of water, it also discards off bacteria for the treatment of urinary tract infections.

Ingredients:

Fresh or dried parsley

Water

Procedure:

Take 1 to 2 cups of water of water in apt. Bring it to boil. Add parsley one cup if fresh and two tablespoons if dried). Reduce the heat of the flame. Boil for 5 to 10 minutes. Take it off the flame. Cool it and strain it into a cup. Your parsley water is ready to drink.

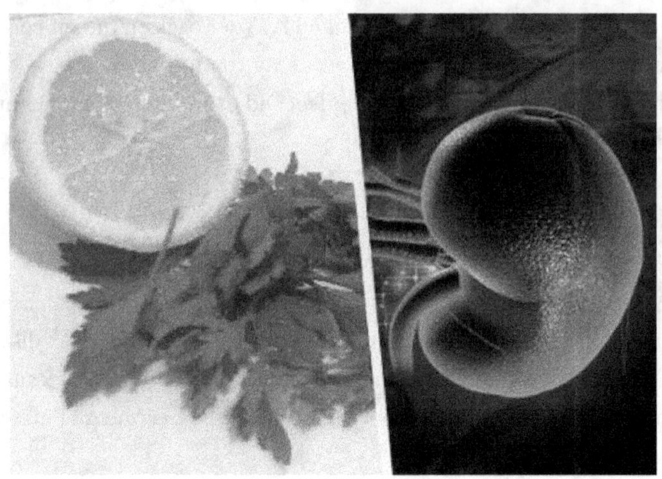

Flu Compress

3 Cups water

25 Drops Lavender Essential oil

25 Drops Peppermint essential oil

2 tbsp Thyme

2 tbsp Feverfew

- Boil the herbs in the water

- Add the essential oils

- Damp a clean cloth

- Place cloth on forehead

- Replace cloth when cool.

Licorice Root

The licorice is a plant and its roots are used to make medicine. It is used to flavor foods, beverages, and tobacco. If you are suffering from digestive system problems, then you can use it because it is perfect to treat colic, stomach ulcers, and heartburn. It is also beneficial to use for constant gastritis. It is also useful for the infections of bacteria, including cough, bronchitis, and sore throat.

You can use it for liver disorders, malaria, CFS (chronic fatigue syndrome), food poisoning and tuberculosis. It can be used with the combination of Panax ginseng and Bupleurum falciparum to enhance its benefits. It is important to produce essential hormones that enable your body to response stress.

If you want to increase the fertility of women, then the licorice can be used with another herb known as shakuyaku-kanzo-to. It helps in the treatment of the polycystic ovary syndrome. Sometimes, it is used to treat the oily hair, and it contains several chemicals to decrease the swelling and cough. It can make the mucus secretions thin, and enhance the chemicals in the body requires treating ulcers.

Side Effects of Licorice

- The licorice is used for food and medicinal purposes in larger amounts. Its purpose is to treat different ailments in a short period of time. It can be applied to the skin for a short period of time to heal it.

- It is unsafe to use more than 4 weeks because the long-term consumption of the licorice can be the reason of high blood pressure, paralysis, low potassium levels, brain damage and heart disease. It should not be consumed on a frequent basis to avoid these side effects.

Interactions of the Licorice

The licorice can interact with warfarin because the warfarin is typically used to reduce the blood clotting. The body usually works to break down the warfarin to expel it out from your body. The licorice can increase the breakdown process and reduce its efficiency. You have to check your blood on a regular basis to check the dosage of warfarin.

Dosage of Licorice

If you want to treat an upset stomach, you can treat it with the particular combination of licorice and different other herbs. Take 1 mL three times a day to get its maximum benefits.

Your Mouth

When your mouth is healthy, your body can stave off a lot of infections. When you don't take proper care of your teeth and gums, you can run into problems.

Abscess Wash

1 Cup of Listerine or other unflavored antiseptic mouthwash.

2 Tablespoons Sage

1 tablespoon Echinacea

1 Tablespoon White Oak Bark

35 Drops of Tea Tree oil

- Place all of the ingredients in a jar with a tight lid.

- Shake and place in a dark, cool, place.

- Shake once in the morning and once at night.

- Do this for three days.

- Strain the herbs out.

- Use the normal amount of mouthwash before brushing your teeth.

The Oak Bark and the Sage will pull out the infection. The Tea Tree and Echinacea will kill it. The Sage will also bring down the swelling.

Gingivitis Rub

1/2 Cup of Coconut oil

2 tbsp Sage

1 tbsp Echinacea or Green Tea

10 Drops of Peppermint Essential oil

15 Drops of Lavender Essential oil

- Heat the herbs in the oil overnight in a crock pot

- Using a cheesecloth, strain out the herbs.

- Place the oil in a dark glass container.

- Add the essential oils when the oil is Luke Warm

- Apply to the gums after you have brushed your teeth.

The herbs and essential oils will work together to help bring down swelling and repair the damage to your gums while preventing infections.

Chest congestion

We all get those chest colds. We feel like we can't draw a breath without coughing. Coughing is the body's natural way of getting rid of viruses and infections. It may be gross to think about, but when you cough something up, don't swallow it. Spit it out. It will speed your recovery.

Soda water:

Soda water here does not mean carbonated drinks. Soda water means that it is made up of soda. Soda is an alkaline substance and can decrease the acidity of the urine by making it neutral. This remedy is useful for urinary tract infections and prevents kidney stone formation. If you have a problem in urinating then soda water can be an exquisite tonic in this case. It is also be used for the treatment of heart burn as it also neutralizes the acid in the stomach.

Ingredient:

Baking soda

Water

Procedure:

Take a glass of water. Add one teaspoon of soda in it. Stir it with the spoon till it is dissolved. Your soda water is ready.

Drink it in the mooring before your breakfast. Do not drink for more than a week and if you are avoiding sodium as it contains sufficient quantity of sodium.

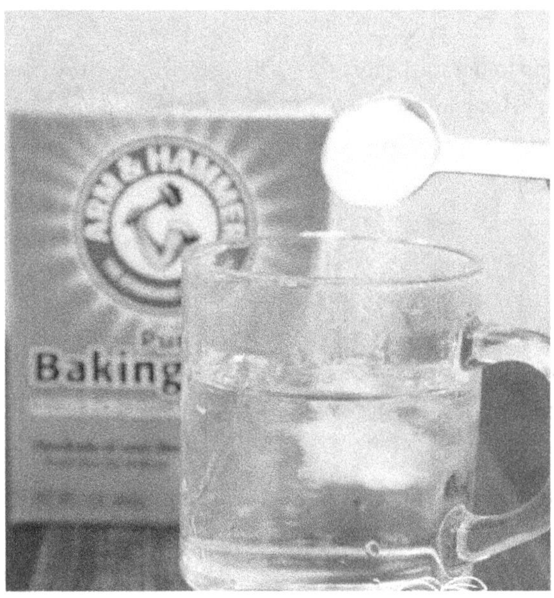

Massaging with Olive oil

Olive oil is best as far as the eating is concern and for the massaging purposes as well. You can massage your joints with it and keep it warm as well. The compounds in the oil makes sure that it lubricates and gets the tissues assembled back to the joints.

Olive oil keeps you moist internally and helps your body retain in the times when you are not able to react much. You cannot just apply every oil on your body and expect it to relieve the pain but olive oil has the natural power to take away the pains. Do not depend on the heavy medications or the pain killers which would be affect only for the time being.

Some people tend to put the heat relieving patches, they are also good but they do not help you get rid of pain for a longer time. The pain would be back within some hours so it is better to massage the area in which you have pain daily with the olive oil and rest for a bit.

The best time to do that is during winters because you do not have any AC on and there is no chance of you getting reacted by any kind of coldness. You do not have to cook or warm the olive. Even if you keep it at a cool place, its affect would be warm which will give you ease.

Make sure to rub it gently without pressing it too hard on your body part because we do not want that you end up getting a sprain or a bruise. Do it gently and keep rubbing the area. The most preferable type of olive oil would be the extra virgin olive oil.

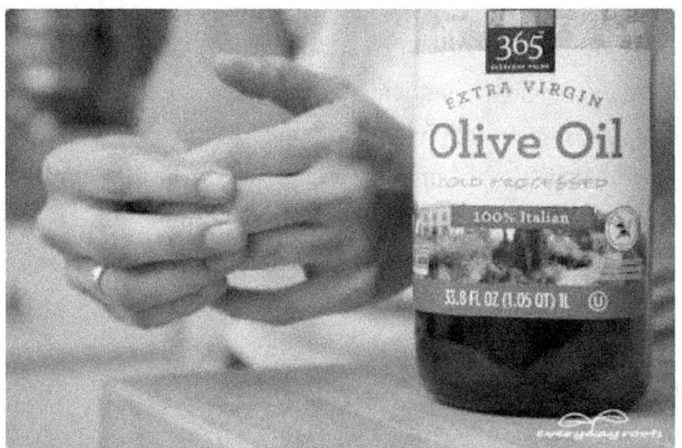

Chest pack

1 Cup hot water

1/2 Fresh Ginger root crushed

2 tbsp Cinnamon

15 Drops Peppermint Essential oil

15 Drops of Lemon Essential oil

- Crush the fresh Ginger in a bowl to retain the juice

- Add the Cinnamon

- Add the Essential oils

- Add just enough of the water to make the paste warm.

- Apply the paste to the chest and cover with plastic wrap.

- When it is completely cool, remove and shower as normal.

Cat's Claw

The Cat's claw is a useful herb to treat stomach problem. It is famous for its exceptional properties to strengthen the immune system of your body. It will enable your body to fight infections and different infections. The oxindole alkaloids can enhance the capacity of the immune system to destroy the pathogens. You can use this herb for the treatment painful and swollen joints, and the 8 weeks are enough to treat different health problems.

Dosage of the Cat's Claw

- You can take one gram of root bark 2 to 3 times a day, and the ideal dosage of the root is 20 to 30 mg. You should not take the products of the cat's claw before surgery and immunosuppressant therapy.

- There can be some adverse reactions of the herb, including stomach pain, diarrhea, and nausea. If you want to avoid the side effects of this herb, then you should take its limited dose. Consult your doctor to know either herb can interact with your current medication.

Cold and Flu Tea

1 pot of water (12 cups)

1 tbsp of Echinacea

1/2 tbsp Ginger

1 tbsp Thyme

1 tbsp Feverfew

1 tbsp Calendula petals

1/2 tbsp Chamomile

- Mix all of the herbs in the coffee filter.

- Brew a pot as normal.

- Sweeten with raw honey

- Add Lemon Juice

- You can also add 5 drops of peppermint essential oil, but that is optional.

Chest Ointment

1/4 Cup of Cayenne Pepper

1/4 cup of fresh Ginger

1/2 cup of Echinacea

1 Cup of Olive oil

1/4 Cup beeswax

25 Drops of Peppermint Essential oil

20 Drops of Lavender Essential oil

10 drops of Tea Tree essential oil

Dark glass jars to store it in

- Place the herbs and oil in a crock pot overnight.

- Use a cheese cloth to strain it out.

- Put the oil back in the double boiler and heat

- Add the beeswax and wait until it melts

- Pour into your containers

- Mix the essential oils

- Add the essential oils when the main mixture is warm and not hot.

- Apply to the chest and under nose as needed to break up sinus and chest pressure.

Egg Whites:

- This one might never have been tried before as a home remedy but it is very famous normally. Put two eggs in a bowl and take aside the egg yellow. Then sink the burn and soak it in egg whites. It really works instantly and the pain may just go forever after a few hours of getting your burn in the egg whites. Try it out, eggs aren't expensive either.

- There is a significantly low information and knowledge in people about how exactly they need to respond in a situation where you've got a cut. We all somewhere in our lives experienced a mishap and we ran here and there thinking about what to do to stop the bleeding. It's a petrifying situation and most people are unable to deal with it since the sight of blood and panic around makes people go blank and have their hearts in their mouth.

- It's usually thought that putting on a bandage would stop the bleeding but what's really important here to note is that the blood flows at a rapid rate and till the time you bring a bandage from a nearby chemist or pharmacy, a lot of spillage would have been done, resulting in a life threatening situation for the person who has gotten the cut.

That's why, it is very essential to know what remedies you can immediately undertake instead of panicking and half-killing the affected person.

Use Ice to Stop Bleeding:

- Put on some cubes of ice on the area where there is a cut. It is a very useful remedy to immediately address bleeding caused by a cut.
- The turmeric powder can also help you to stop the bleeding. As we discussed earlier, the herbal turmeric is very useful in the body whether you eat it or you apply it. Some people are scared that it may leave the color behind but that is okay and it will be washed off once you take shower so do not exempt from it with the fear of its color and keep on bearing the pain or bleed. Simple take the turmeric powder and apply it on the cut or the area where it is bleeding. Within few minutes the bleeding will stop and you will a lot better.
- Cayenne Pepper can be another source to stop the bleeding. Well, the pepper word itself is hurtful but it will better once you are done with it. If you are someone who is scared of bees then consider to keep this pepper with you all the time because it will be needed badly and would be useful as well immediately.

Peppermint tea:

Peppermint acts as a soothing agent. It can ease the stomach pain and gas problems. Menthol which is an essential oil in the peppermint acts as an antispasmodic agent. It also has effects that allow to sooth nerves thus, relieving stomach pain. You can drink this tea after dinner which will help you to digest food readily.

Method 1:

Ingredients:

Peppermint tea (tea bag)

Water

Honey (if required)

Lemon (if necessary)

Procedure:

Take a cup of water in a pan. Heat it till it gets boiled. Put the tea bag in the cup. Pour the piping hot water in the cup. Cover the cup with a lid or small plate. Let it be there for 15 minutes. Move the tea bag up and down, and your peppermint tea is ready to be used. You can also add honey or lemon for taste.

Method 2:

Ingredients:

Peppermint leaves

Fennel

Cardamom

Water

Honey (if required)

Lemon (if required)

Method:

Take a cup of water in a pot. Heat it till its boil. Add peppermint leaves, Fennel, cardamom in it. Give it boil for two times. Strain it into a cup. Let it e cool a little. Your peppermint tea is ready to be used. You can also add honey or lemon for taste.

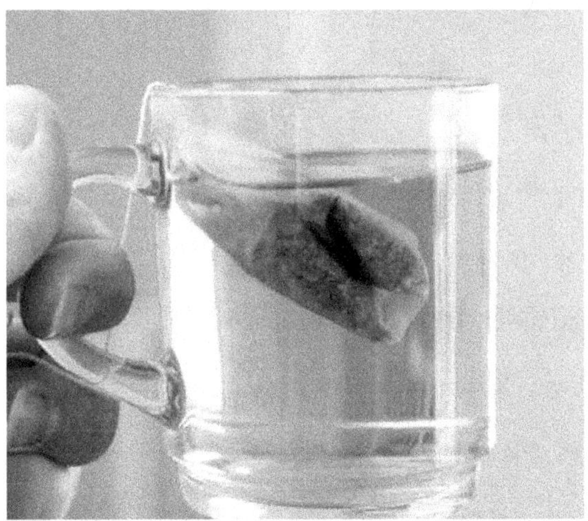

Cold and Flu Bath

1/4 Cup Fine Sea Salt

1/4 Cup Epsom Salt

1/4 Cup Baking Soda

1/8 Cup Borax

3 tbsp ground fresh ginger

2 tbsp Rosemary leaves, ground

3 tbsp ground Echinacea

1/4 Cup Olive oil

10 Drops Peppermint

10 Drops Lavender Essential oil

5 Drops Tea Tree oil

- Add all the dry ingredients first.

- Mix all the oils separately

- Slowly add the oil to the dry ingredients.

- Mix well and place in an air-tight container

- Leave it sit overnight.

- Add 1/4 Cup to running water

Cabbage

The cabbage is an important member of the cruciferous family of vegetables, including cauliflower, kale, broccoli and sprouts. The cabbage is famous for its healing power because the sulfur compounds in the cabbage are ideal to treat cancer. It is high in vitamin C, and one cup of cabbage may serve as a natural antibiotic.

Procedure to Use Cabbage

A cup of fresh cabbage juice 2 to 3 times a day will help you to treat stomach ulcers. You can add a half teaspoon of honey in the cabbage juice to enhance its taste. You can chew raw cabbage to get its enzymes. The leaves of raw cabbage may help you to treat tender breasts and inflammation caused by the mastitis and fibro cysts.

Garlic

If you want to look for ways on how to some treat bacterial infection, then you should not skip any ginger effect, which is very efficient in treating factors like stomach infection and other respiratory disease.

Procedure to Use Garlic

It helps to cool down your body and boost your blood circulation at the same time. As a result, the ginger effect will help you to reduce the amount of all the bad bacteria in your body. To treat and cure your respiratory infection, it is also highly recommended that you are drinking ginger at least tea 3-4 times during a day.

Moreover, you can always massage your affected skin by garlic pieces. By boosting all the blood circulation, this is the way we will help you reduce the pain that is caused by bacterial infection.

Ginger extract can always be used for the massaging on the affected areas of the body for the treating bacterial infections and for controlling all the pain. For instance, take a stalk of ginger on every day to prevent infections of all the body.

Flaxseed oil:

Flaxseed oil is easily available at the grocery stores. It is usually used for relieving constipation. It increases the number of bowel movements in a day. You can add orange with it as it will taste better and also orange has fiber in it which increases the roughage and soften the stools.

Ingredients:

Orange juice with pulp

Flaxseed oil

Procedure:

Take one glass of orange juice with its pulp. Add one tablespoon of flax seed oil. Drink this mixture. This remedy will open your bowel within 5 hours so, wait till then and avoid unnecessary repetition.

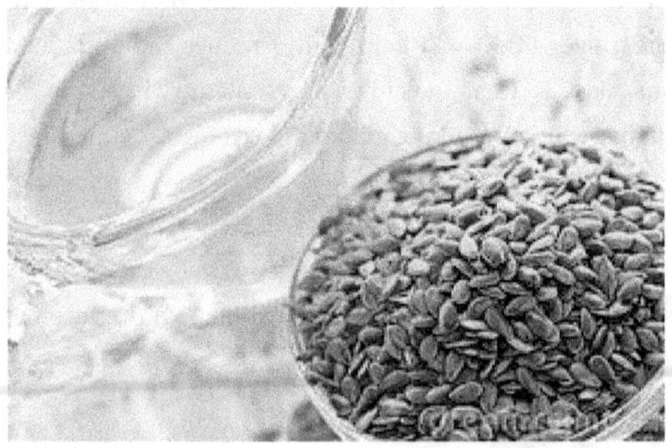

Cinnamon tea:

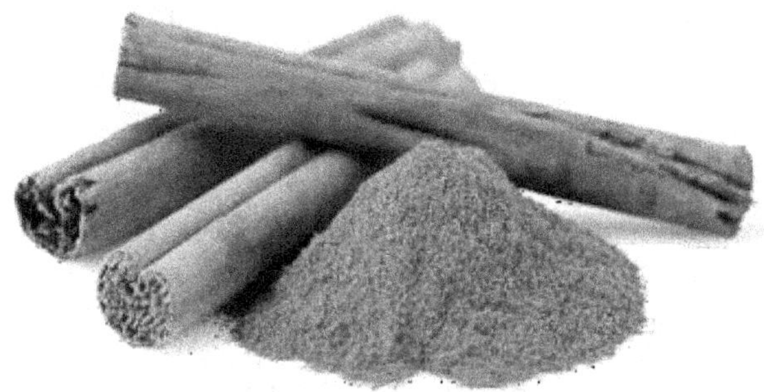

Cinnamon is readily available and can be used for the treatment of vomiting. Whenever you feel nausea or having to vomit then, cinnamon tea is the remedy of choice.

Ingredients:

Cinnamon sticks or powder

Water

Honey

Procedure:

Take a cup of water. Pour it in a pot. Boil the water. Add one teaspoon of cinnamon into it. If you do not have cinnamon powder, then you can also use a cinnamon stick. Give two or three boils. Take it off the flame. Allow it to relay for 10 minutes. Strain it with the help of a strainer. Your cinnamon tea is ready for drinking. You can also add honey for taste.

Lavender flower tea:

Lavender can be used as an ornamental purpose or for medicinal use. It is also used for the treatment of anxiety and insomnia.

Ingredients:

Lavender flowers (fresh or dried)

Water

Procedure:

For a relaxing, yourself of anxiety pour some of the lavender flowers in the water and take a bath from it. It will relieve your anxiety.

For a restful sleep, put some fresh flowers or pouch of dried flower of lavender under your pillow. It will allow you to sleep calmly.

Tart cherry juice:

Tart cherry juice can be one of the remedies that can help you sleep in the night. It contains tryptophan. Tryptophan is an essential amino acid that is converted to serotonin in the body which in turn is converted to melatonin. Melatonin helps to regulate sleep and its pattern.

Ingredients:

Tart cherries

Water

Procedure:

Take few tart cherries and put them in the blender. Blend this mixture till a smooth paste is formed. Add a small amount of water to increase the consistency. Take half or one glass of this juice.

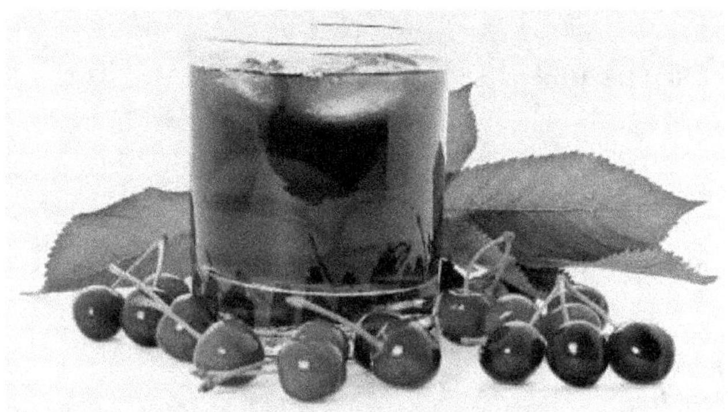

Burn ointment

1/2 Cup Olive oil

1/4 cup Beeswax

1/4 Cup Calendula petals

25 Drops of Lavender essential oil

- Place the oil and herb in a crock pot overnight

- Use a cheesecloth to strain out the herb

- Reheat the oil in a double boiler

- Melt the beeswax

- Add the mixture to a jar with a tight lid.

- Wait until it is Luke Warm to add the Lavender

- Use on the burn area

Quick fix burn treatment

1 tbsp Aloe gel

6 drops Lavender essential oil

- Mix and apply to burn area

Wound wash

Let's face it. If you have kids, you're going to need a better, and faster way, to clean out a cut or scrape when they come home battered from a day outside or at the park. They're kids, and they play hard.

4 Ounces of warm water

25 Drops of Peppermint Essential oil

25 Drops of Tea Tree Essential oil

4-ounce squirt bottle

- Place all the ingredients in the bottle and shake vigorously

- Squirt into the wound

That's it. It will not only wash the dirt of, or out, it will also disinfect the wound.

Lemon balm:

Lemon balm has been used for so long for the treatment of insomnia and anxiety. It enhances mood and promotes calmness. It contains serotonin that is converted into melatonin.

Ingredients:

Lemon balm

Water

Honey

Chamomile flower

Procedure:

Take a cup of water in a pot and heat it. Turn off the heat. Put the lemon balm and chamomile flowers in the pot. Add hot water into the cup and cover the pot with the lid. Strain the tea in a cup. You can also add honey fro taste.

Saint John's wort tea:

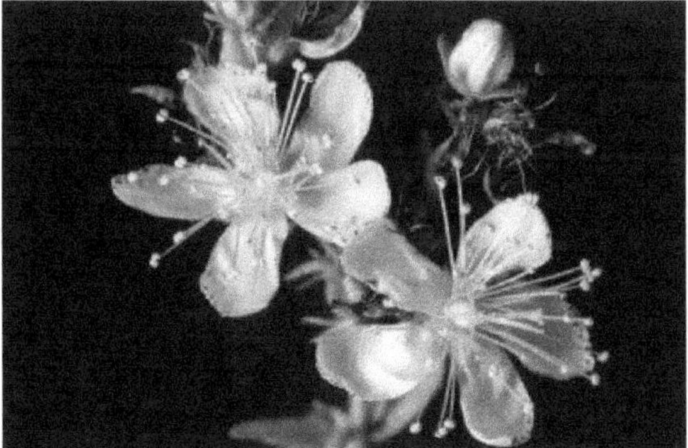

Saint John's main component is hypericin. Hypercine is a reuptake in inhibitor of serotonin and increases serotonin level in the brain. Serotonin is then converted into melatonin which helps in regulating sleep. It is also used for calmness and reduces anxiety.

Ingredients:

Saint John's wort

Water

Honey (if required)

Lemon juice (if required)

Procedure:

Take a cup of water in a pot and boil it. Add two teaspoon of Saint John's wort into it. Rinse the mixture in a cup with the help of the strainer. You can also add lemon juice or honey for enhancing its taste.

Bruise ointment

1/2 Cup of Olive oil

1/4 Beeswax

1/4 Cup Marjoram

1/4 Cup Echinacea

- Steep the herbs overnight in a crock pot on low.

- Use a cheesecloth to strain them out.

- Reheat the oil in a double boiler

- Melt the Beeswax

- Add the ointment to dark glass jars.

- Wait until it cools.

- Apply to bruises.

Milk:

Milk can be used for treating insomnia. It contains serotonin which is converted into melatonin in the body. Melatonin helps to regulate sleep pattern of the body. It also increases internal body temperature that helps you to sleep. It also has some psychological effect that allows you to sleep calmly.

Ingredients:

Milk

Honey (if required)

Procedure:

Take a glass of milk in a pot and heat it till it's slightly warm. Pour this milk in a cup. You can also add honey to it for taste. Drink this milk 30 minutes before going to bed.

First aid ointment

1 Cup of Olive oil

1/2 Cup of Beeswax

1/4 Cup of Sage

4 Large Bay leaves

1/4 Cup of Marjoram

1/4 Cup of Calendula Petals

1/4 Cup of Echinacea

20 Drops of Lavender Essential oil

20 Drops of Peppermint Essential oil

10 Drops of Tea Tree Oil

- Steep the herbs overnight in a crock pot on low

- Using a cheesecloth, strain out the herbs

- Place the oil in a double boiler

- Melt the beeswax into the olive oil

- Mix the essential oils.

- Place the ointment into dark glass jars.

- When it is Luke Warm, add equal amounts of the essential oil blend

- Apply to cuts, scrapes, bruises or other wounds.

- You can even apply it to bandage and then the wound.

For bad breath:

Many of us encounter bad breath. This bad breath can be because of many problems in the digestive system. It can be due to a problem affecting our teeth, tonsils or any part of the digestive tract. This bad breath can produce a bad impression of a person. Here we are giving you a home remedy that can help you with getting rid of this bad breath. Parsley has its effect that allows a person to get rid of the bad breath.

Method 1:

Ingredients:

Parsley

Procedure:

It is a very simple process to follow. All you need is to take a small amount of parsley and chew it directly.

Method 2:

Ingredients:

Parsley

Vinegar

Procedure:

Take a cup of parsley and dip it in a bowl of vinegar. Keep it for few hours. Take the parsley and then chew them whenever you feel your breath is not good.

Method 3:

Ingredients:

Parsley

Water

Procedure:

Take a cup of parsley. Put the leaves in the blender. Blend the leaves and add a cup of water. Drink this juice whenever you need to get rid of bad breath.

Herbal bath for sprains

Depending on whether it's your back or a smaller part of the body, you will need to scale it appropriately.

1 ounce of Marjoram

1 ounce of Bay leaves

Reusable filter bag

- Place the herbs in the bag

- Place the bag in a tub of running hot water

- Swirl the water around before laying the tub.

- Soak the sprained body part.

- you can scale it down to coffee pot size by doing the following:

- o   3 coffee scoops of Marjoram

- o   4 bay leaves

- o   Brew like it's coffee

- o   Add to a foot soak for feet, elbows or ankles.

Mineral Foot Soak

Achy feet need love, too. They carry us hither and yon without a complaint, most of the time.

1/4 Cup Sea salt, fine

1/4 Cup Epsom Salt

1/4 cup baking soda

1/8 cup Olive oil

1/8 cup Ground sage

10 Drops Peppermint Oil

10 Drops Lavender oil

- Mix all the dry ingredient and set them aside

- Mix all the oils well

- Slowly add the oils to the dry ingredients

- Place in an air-tight container overnight.

- Add 1/8 cup to warm water in a foot soak/massager.

Tight and achy muscle rub

After a long day of stooping, lifting, and moving around, your back may feel tight, strained and even hurt. A good massage oil will do the trick.

Word to the wise: Do NOT massage pulled muscles. You will make them worse.

1 Cup Olive oil

1/4 cup Black Pepper

1/4 cup sage

1/4 Cup Allspice

1/4 Echinacea

25 Drops of Lavender essential oil

25 Drops of Peppermint

- Steep the herbs in the oil in a crock pot overnight

- Strain out the herbs

- Wait until the oil cools to add the essential oils

- Mix well

- Massage into the tight muscles.

- You can even add this to the base mineral bath mixture above for a nice relaxing bath.

- You can even make this mixture into an ointment to rub into smaller areas like knees and elbows.

Quick and dirty remedies

- 1 tsp of Baking soda in a 1/4 cup of warm water can alleviate a case of heartburn.

- Adding three drops of peppermint essential oil to a cotton ball and placing it on a heating vent in your car can ease you tension on the ride home.

- Putting 50 drops of Lemon essential oil in your rinse water can sanitize surfaces as you clean.

- Making onion oil and putting a few drops in your ear can alleviate an ear ache.

- One teaspoon of Apple Cider Vinegar in a 1/4 cup of warm water can dry up weeping eczema and psoriasis.

- Putting used Green Tea bags on your eyes can help with wrinkles and bags around the eye area.

- Making cucumber oil from the skin can tighten skin and help clear up acne.

- Cucumber juice added to Witch Hazel is a great base for a facial astringent.

- Adding two drops of Lavender Essential oil to your baby's soap relaxes them and helps them sleep.

- Adding six drops of Lavender essential oil to a candle warmer in a baby's room can help them sleep soundly.

- Adding ten drops of Lavender essential oil to a candle warmer in an adult's room can allay anxiety and help you fall asleep faster.

- Adding 1/4 tsp of Tea tree oil to a bowl of warm water can kill fleas when you dunk a flea comb in it.

- Making a tea with cloves and placing it in a spray bottle can be an effective bug repellant. Spray it on lawn furniture and even on your pets.

- Adding Peppermint essential oil to baking soda can kill fleas in the carpet. Just mix 10 drops per two tablespoons of baking soda. Wait until it's dry before you sprinkle in your carpet. Work it into your carpet, and then vacuum it up. You can use 5 drops of Tea Tree and Five drops of Peppermint essential oils for a double punch.

Conclusion

People are turning to natural remedies aka home remedies, or natural cures, for their ailments or other diseases because these treatments are entirely made with natural ingredients such as fruits, herbs, and vegetables. All ingredients that maybe readily found at home are the reason why people prefer natural remedies.

Home remedies do not always promote the use of harsh chemicals that are inexpensive and usually do not produce any side effects, whatsoever. People also enjoy making something very useful to use instead of paying some expensive over-the-counter drugs that can have very dangerous side effects.

Humans throughout the history have relied on natural remedies before the invention of modern medicine and other synthetic drugs. Most common ailments have known to be treatments with ingredients that are found in your kitchen. Researchers have also discovered that thousands of healing nutrients in the foods are those that we eat every day.

Therefore, through this book, an attempt has been made to help create awareness among people about the brilliant use of natural remedies that could help in every way possible and cure all the deadly and the routine based diseases, viruses, and infections.